DENTAL HEALTH COOKBOOKS FOR KIDS

"Grin & Cook: A Recipe Book for Healthy Teeth and Happy Kids"

Harold L. Robinson

1

Introduction

Dental Health Cookbooks for Kids: A Mouthwatering Introduction

Children's oral health is vital for their general health and well-being. Strong teeth and gums help youngsters eat correctly, talk clearly, and smile boldly. But with so many sugary snacks and beverages accessible, it may be tough for parents to make sure their kids are eating a nutritious diet that's excellent for their teeth.

That's where dental health cookbooks for kids come in. These cookbooks provide a selection of tasty and healthy recipes that are particularly intended to encourage excellent dental health. They also educate youngsters about the significance of dental hygiene and how to care for their teeth and gums.

One of the nicest things about dental health cookbooks for kids is that they make healthy eating enjoyable. With recipes for anything from fruity smoothies and yoghurt parfaits to vegetarian burgers and creamy baked potatoes, kids are sure to find something they love to eat. And since the recipes are simple to follow, even the youngest cooks may get engaged in the kitchen.

In addition to being tasty and healthy, dental health cookbooks for kids may also be a terrific method to educate youngsters about the significance of oral cleanliness. Many of these recipes feature amusing information about teeth and gums, as well as recommendations on how to brush and floss effectively. And by getting kids involved in making nutritious meals and snacks, parents may help them build good eating habits that will last a lifetime.

Here are just a handful of the numerous advantages of utilising dental health recipes for kids:

Teach students about the significance of dental hygiene. Dental health cookbooks may educate youngsters about the numerous kinds of food that are excellent for their teeth and gums, as well as how to brush and floss correctly. This understanding may help kids prevent cavities and other oral issues down the line.

Promote good eating habits. Dental health cookbooks provide a selection of tasty and healthy recipes that are particularly intended to enhance excellent dental health. By consuming these foods, kids may acquire the nutrients they need for healthy teeth and gums, as well as their general health and well-being.

Make healthy eating entertaining. Dental health cookbooks generally offer colourful and entertaining recipes that kids are guaranteed to adore. This may make healthy eating more pleasurable and motivating for youngsters.

Get youngsters engaged in the kitchen. Dental health cookbooks are a terrific way to get youngsters engaged in the kitchen. By helping to create nutritious meals and snacks, kids may learn about various foods and culinary skills. They may also acquire a feeling of success and pride in their culinary talents.

If you're searching for a strategy to encourage healthy eating habits and excellent oral health in your kids, dental health cookbooks are a terrific alternative. With their tasty recipes, amusing information, and helpful recommendations, these cookbooks may make a great impact on your child's overall health and well-being.

Chapter 1

What is dental health?

Dental health is the status of your teeth, gums, and the overall oral-facial system that enables you to smile, talk, and chew. It comprises psychological characteristics such as self-confidence, well-being, and the capacity to interact and work without pain, discomfort, or shame.

Good oral health is vital for individuals of all ages, but it is particularly critical for children. Children's teeth are still growing, and they are more sensitive to cavities and other dental disorders than adult teeth. Additionally, children with poor oral health are more likely to have issues with eating, speaking, and learning.

There are a variety of things you can do to maintain excellent oral health, including:

- Teeth should be brushed twice daily with fluoride toothpaste.

- Flossing your teeth once a day

- Eating a healthy diet

- Avoiding sugary drinks

- Seeing your dentist for regular checkups and cleanings

If you have any concerns regarding your oral health, be sure to speak to your dentist. They can help you spot any possible concerns and build a strategy to maintain your teeth and gums healthy.

Here are some further facts regarding the significance of oral health and how to preserve it:

Strong teeth and gums are crucial for optimal nutrition. They help us chew food correctly so that we can get the nutrients we need.

Dental health is very crucial for our general health. Studies have indicated that those with poor oral health are more likely to have other health concerns, such as heart disease, stroke, and diabetes.

A healthy grin may increase our confidence and self-esteem. It may also make it simpler to mingle and engage with people.

There are a variety of activities you can do to maintain excellent oral health at home, including:

Teeth should be brushed twice daily with fluoride toothpaste. Be careful to brush all surfaces of your teeth, including the front, rear, and top.

Floss your teeth once a day. Flossing helps eliminate plaque and food particles from between your teeth, where your toothbrush can't reach.

Eat a healthy diet. Avoid sugary meals and beverages, which may lead to cavities.

Drink lots of water. Water helps keep your mouth wet and avoids dry mouth, which may contribute to cavities and gum disease.

It is also necessary to visit your dentist for regular exams and cleanings. Your dentist may check your teeth and gums for indicators of abnormalities, such as cavities, gum disease, and oral cancer. They can also clean your teeth and remove plaque and tartar that you can't remove on your own.

By following these easy steps, you may maintain excellent oral health for a lifetime.

How this cookbook can benefit your child's dental health

This cookbook is particularly developed to assist encourage excellent oral health in youngsters. It features a selection of tasty and healthy meals that are cooked using items that are beneficial for teeth and gums. The cookbook also educates youngsters about the significance of dental hygiene and how to care for their teeth and gums appropriately.

Here are some of the ways that this cookbook may assist your child's oral health:

- **Teach students about the significance of dental hygiene:** The cookbook contains entertaining information about teeth and gums, as well as suggestions on how to clean and floss correctly. This information may help youngsters prevent cavities and other oral issues down the line.

- **Promote good eating habits:** The cookbook includes a selection of tasty and healthy dishes that are particularly tailored to encourage excellent dental health. By consuming these foods, kids may acquire the nutrients they need for healthy teeth and gums, as well as their general health and well-being.

- **Make healthy eating entertaining:** The cookbook features colourful and fascinating recipes that kids are likely to adore. This may make healthy eating more pleasurable and motivating for youngsters.

- **Get youngsters engaged in the kitchen:** The cookbook is a terrific way to get youngsters interested in the kitchen. By helping to create nutritious meals and snacks, kids may learn about various foods and culinary skills. They may also acquire a feeling of success and pride in their culinary talents.

In addition to these advantages, the cookbook may also assist to:

Reduce your child's risk of cavities. The dishes in the cookbook are low in sugar and acid, which may lead to cavities.

Improve your child's gum health. The dishes in the cookbook contain foods that are rich in vitamins and minerals that are needed for excellent gum health.

Boost your child's overall health. The dishes in the cookbook are cooked using nutrient-rich ingredients that are helpful for general health and well-being.

By following this cookbook, you can help your kid establish healthy eating habits and excellent dental health that will last a lifetime.

Here are some particular examples of how the dishes in this cookbook might assist your child's oral health:

- **Fruit smoothies:** Fruit smoothies are a terrific way to receive your child's daily dosage of fruits and veggies. Fruits and vegetables are rich with vitamins, minerals, and antioxidants that are needed for optimum oral health.
- **Yoghurt parfaits:** Yogurt parfaits are a delightful and healthy snack that is beneficial for teeth and gums. Yogurt is a rich source of calcium, which is vital for healthy teeth.
- **Veggie burgers:** Veggie burgers are a healthier alternative to regular hamburgers. They are created with veggies, legumes, and grains, which are all beneficial for teeth and gums.
- **Cheesy baked potatoes:** Cheesy baked potatoes are a comfort dish that may also be excellent for teeth and

gums. Potatoes are an excellent source of potassium, which is crucial for keeping healthy gums.

By picking dishes from this cookbook, you can be confident that your kid is receiving the nutrients they need for optimal oral health.

Chapter 2

Using food to promote oral health

Food may play a significant role in supporting oral health. Eating a balanced diet that includes foods that are beneficial for teeth and gums may help avoid cavities, gum disease, and other dental issues.

Here are some strategies for utilising food to boost dental health:

- **Eat lots of fruits and vegetables:** Fruits and vegetables are rich with vitamins, minerals, and antioxidants that are needed for optimal dental health. For example, vitamin C is vital for keeping healthy gums, while calcium is important for strong teeth.
- **Choose whole grains over processed grains:** Whole grains are a wonderful source of fibre, which may assist to clean teeth and gums. Refined

grains, on the other hand, are less nutritious and may lead to plaque accumulation.

- **Limit sugary meals and beverages:** Sugar is a primary food source for bacteria in the mouth. When bacteria devour sugar, they generate acids that may harm teeth and contribute to cavities.
- **Drink lots of water:** Water helps to keep the mouth wet and avoids dry mouth, which may lead to cavities and gum disease.

Here are some particular examples of foods that are helpful for dental health:

- **Dairy products:** Dairy products are a rich source of calcium, which is vital for healthy teeth.
- **Fruits and veggies:** Fruits and vegetables are filled with vitamins, minerals, and antioxidants that are needed for optimum dental health.

Some healthy selections are apples, carrots, celery, leafy green vegetables, berries, and citrus fruits.

- **Whole grains:** Whole grains are a wonderful source of fibre, which may assist to clean teeth and gums. Some healthful alternatives are brown rice, quinoa, and oats.
- **Nuts and seeds:** Nuts and seeds are a wonderful source of calcium, phosphorus, and vitamin D, which are all vital for healthy dental health. Some healthy options are almonds, cashews, peanuts, and sunflower seeds.
- **Lean protein:** Lean protein foods, such as chicken, fish, and beans, are rich providers of phosphorus, which is needed for healthy teeth.

In addition to eating a healthy diet, there are a few more things you can do to utilise food to boost oral health:

- **Chew sugar-free gum after meals:** Chewing sugar-free gum may assist stimulate saliva production, which can help wash away food particles and microorganisms.
- **Eat crunchy foods:** Crunchy foods, such as apples, carrots, and celery, may aid in cleaning teeth and gums.
- **Avoid sticky foods:** Sticky foods, such as sweets and taffy, may adhere to teeth and contribute to cavities.

By following these guidelines, you may utilise food to promote excellent dental health for yourself and your family.

15 kid-friendly recipes to promote dental health (Age 2 and above)

Here are 15 kid-friendly recipes that enhance oral health (age 2 and above):

Breakfast

- **Oatmeal with berries and nuts:** This is an excellent source of fibre, which helps to clean teeth and gums. The berries and nuts also give crucial vitamins and minerals that are helpful for oral health.
- **Yoghurt parfait:** This is a fantastic source of calcium, protein, and fibre. Calcium is vital for healthy teeth, protein helps to repair and rebuild gum tissue, and fibre helps to clean teeth and gums.
- **Smoothie:** Smoothies are a terrific method to encourage youngsters to eat their fruits and veggies. They are also a wonderful source of calcium,

protein, and vitamins, which are all vital for oral health.

Lunch

- **Veggie quesadillas:** These are wonderful sources of fibre and vitamins, which are all vital for tooth health. They are also a fun and quick snack for youngsters to enjoy.
- **Chicken nuggets:** These are a rich source of protein, which is vital for repairing and rebuilding gum tissue. They are also quite low in sugar, which is helpful for tooth health.
- **Fruit and yoghurt parfait:** This is a fantastic source of calcium, protein, and fibre. Calcium is vital for healthy teeth, protein helps to repair and rebuild gum tissue, and fibre helps to clean teeth and gums.

Dinner

- **Salmon with roasted vegetables:** Salmon is an excellent source of omega-3 fatty acids, which are helpful for general health, including tooth health. Roasted veggies are a wonderful source of fibre and vitamins, which are also vital for tooth health.
- **Chicken stir-fry:** Chicken stir-fry is a fast and simple dish that is filled with nutrition. Chicken is a rich source of protein, which is vital for repairing and rebuilding gum tissue. Vegetables are a wonderful source of fibre and vitamins, which are also vital for oral health.
- **Lentil soup:** Lentil soup is a substantial and healthy meal that is helpful for oral health. Lentils are a wonderful source of fibre and protein, which are vital for tooth health. Vegetables are a wonderful source of

fibre and vitamins, which are also vital for oral health.

Snacks

- **Trail mix:** Trail mix is a wonderful source of protein, fibre, and healthy fats, which are all necessary for oral health. It is also a handy snack that is convenient to carry on the run.
- **Hard-boiled eggs:** Hard-boiled eggs are a wonderful source of protein, which is vital for repairing and rebuilding gum tissue. They are also a handy snack that is convenient to carry on the run.
- **Fruit and veggie platter:** This is a fun and nutritious snack choice for youngsters. Be sure to include a variety of fruits and veggies to ensure that your kid is receiving the nutrients they need.
- **Cheese sticks:**Cheese is a rich source of calcium, which is needed for

healthy teeth. Cheese sticks are a practical and portable snack choice for youngsters.

- **Whole-wheat crackers with peanut butter:** Peanut butter is a fantastic source of protein, which is vital for repairing and rebuilding gum tissue. Whole-wheat crackers are a wonderful source of fibre, which helps to clean teeth and gums.

These are just a few examples of kid-friendly recipes that enhance oral health. There are many more fantastic recipes accessible online and in cookbooks. When picking recipes, be careful to consider your child's nutritional requirements and preferences. You may also be creative and experiment with other tastes and ingredients.

Here are some extra recommendations for creating nutritious meals and snacks for kids:

- **Avoid sugary beverages and snacks:** Sugar is the major food supply for bacteria in the mouth, which may lead to cavities.
- Choose water or unsweetened milk instead of sugary beverages.
- **Offer a choice of nutritious meals and snacks:** This will assist to ensure that your kid is receiving the nutrients they need for oral health and general wellness.
- **Be an excellent role model.** Set a good example by eating nutritious meals and snacks yourself.

By following these recommendations, you may help your kid establish good eating habits that will last a lifetime.

Vitamins and minerals

Vitamins and minerals are important chemicals that our bodies need in modest doses to work correctly. They play a role in a vast array of physiological operations, including metabolism, energy production, cell formation and repair, and immune function.

Vitamins are organic substances, which means they are created by plants or animals. Minerals are inorganic elements, which means they come from the ground and water.

There are 13 essential vitamins:

- Vitamin A
- Vitamin C
- Vitamin D
- Vitamin E
- Vitamin K

The B vitamins are as follows: Thiamine Riboflavin Niacin Pantothenic acid Biotin Pyridoxine Folate Cobalamin

There are 16 significant minerals:

- Calcium
- Chloride
- Chromium
- Copper
- Iodine
- Iron
- Magnesium
- Manganese
- Molybdenum
- Nickel
- Phosphorus
- Potassium
- Selenium
- Sodium
- Sulphur
- Zinc

Vitamins and minerals may be obtained via the foods we eat. However, some persons may need to take supplements to acquire enough of certain vitamins and minerals, especially if they have a medical condition or are following a restrictive diet.

Here are some examples of the vital tasks that vitamins and minerals play in our bodies:

- Vitamin A is required for vision, immunological function, and cell formation.

- Vitamin C plays a vital role in the immune system, wound healing and collagen production.

- Vitamin D is vital for bone health, immunological function, and cell formation.

- Vitamin E is an antioxidant that protects cells from injury.

- Vitamin K is extremely vital for blood coagulation and bone health.

B vitamins are vital for energy synthesis, metabolism, and cell function.

- Calcium is vital for bone health, muscle function, and neuron function.

- Chloride is crucial for fluid balance and blood pressure regulation.

- Chromium is crucial for blood sugar regulation.

- Copper is necessary for red blood cell production and iron absorption.
- Iodine is necessary for thyroid function.

- Iron is necessary for red blood cell production and oxygen transport.

- Magnesium is necessary for muscle function, neuron function, and blood pressure regulation.

- Manganese is crucial for bone health and metabolism.

- Molybdenum is vital for metabolism and detoxification.

- Nickel is crucial for enzyme function and cell growth.

- Phosphorus is vital for bone health, energy production, and cell function.

- Potassium is important for fluid balance, blood pressure regulation, and muscle function.

- Selenium is an antioxidant that protects cells from injury.

- Sodium is crucial for fluid balance and blood pressure regulation.

- Sulphur is crucial for protein synthesis and detoxification.

- Zinc is crucial for the immune function, cell growth, and wound healing.

Getting appropriate vitamins and minerals is crucial for good health. Eating a healthy diet that includes a diversity of fruits, vegetables, whole grains, and lean protein is the best way to acquire the vitamins and minerals you need. However, some persons may need to take supplements to acquire enough of certain vitamins and minerals, especially if they have a medical condition or are following a restrictive diet.

whether you are unclear whether you are taking enough vitamins and minerals, talk to your doctor. They can help you examine your needs and recommend the best plan to acquire the nutrients you need.

Food that are good for teeth

Eating a balanced diet is vital for general health, including dental health. There are a variety of foods that are beneficial for teeth, and including them in your diet may help to avoid cavities, gum disease, and other dental issues.

Here are some of the healthiest meals for teeth:

- **Dairy products:** Dairy products are a rich source of calcium, which is vital for healthy teeth. Good options include milk, cheese, and yoghurt.
- **Fruits and vegetables:** Fruits and vegetables are filled with vitamins, minerals, and antioxidants that are needed for optimal oral health. Some healthy selections are apples, carrots, celery, leafy green vegetables, berries, and citrus fruits.
- **Whole grains:** Whole grains are a wonderful source of fibre, which may

assist to clean teeth and gums. Good alternatives include brown rice, quinoa, and oats.

- **Nuts and seeds:** Nuts and seeds are a wonderful source of calcium, phosphorus, and vitamin D, which are all vital for healthy dental health. Good selections include almonds, cashews, peanuts, and sunflower seeds.
- **Lean protein:** Lean protein foods, such as chicken, fish, and beans, are rich providers of phosphorus, which is needed for healthy teeth.

In addition to consuming these foods, there are a few more things you can do to maintain your teeth healthy:

- Teeth should be brushed twice daily with fluoride toothpaste.
- Floss your teeth once a day.
- Always visit your dentist for routine checkups and cleanings.

Here are some particular instances of how the foods mentioned above might improve your teeth:

Dairy products: The calcium in dairy products helps to strengthen the enamel, which is the outer coating of the tooth.

- **Fruits and vegetables:** The vitamins, minerals, and antioxidants in fruits and vegetables help to protect teeth and gums from damage. For example, vitamin C is vital for keeping healthy gums, while calcium is important for strong teeth.
- **Whole grains:** The fibre in whole grains helps to clean teeth and gums by eliminating food particles and plaque.
- **Nuts and seeds:** The calcium, phosphorus, and vitamin D in nuts and seeds are all important for good oral health. Calcium helps to strengthen tooth enamel, phosphorus

helps to form new tooth enamel, and vitamin D helps the body absorb calcium.

- **Lean protein:**The phosphorus in lean protein sources is important for strong teeth. Phosphorus helps form new tooth enamel and keeps teeth strong.

By eating a healthy diet that includes foods that are good for teeth, you can help to keep your teeth healthy and strong for a lifetime.

Food to avoid

There are a number of items that you should avoid or restrict in your diet to safeguard your oral health. These foods may lead to cavities, gum disease, and other dental issues.

Here are some of the top foods to avoid for excellent oral health:

- **Sugary meals and drinks:** Sugar is the major food source for bacteria in the mouth. When bacteria devour sugar, they generate acids that may harm teeth and contribute to cavities. Sugary meals and beverages to avoid include sweets, cookies, cakes, soda, juice, and sports drinks.
- **Starchy foods:** Starchy meals, such as bread, pasta, and rice, may break down into sugar in the mouth. This may lead to cavities. It is advisable to consume starchy foods as part of a

balanced diet and to wash your teeth afterwards.

- **Acidic meals and beverages:** Acidic foods and drinks may erode tooth enamel, rendering teeth more sensitive to cavities. Acidic foods and beverages to avoid include citrus fruits, juices, and sodas.
- **Sticky foods:** Sticky foods, such as sweets, taffy, and caramels, may adhere to teeth and contribute to cavities. It is better to avoid sticky foods completely or to rinse your teeth shortly after eating them.
- **Hard foods:** Hard foods, such as ice, nuts, and hard sweets, may harm teeth and chip or break fillings. It is better to avoid hard meals or to consume them with care.

In addition to avoiding these items, it is also vital to adopt excellent oral hygiene routines, such as brushing your teeth twice a day and flossing once a day. Seeing your dentist for frequent examinations and cleanings is very vital for maintaining excellent oral health.

Here are some recommendations for lowering your consumption of foods that are unhealthy for your teeth:

- **Choose water over sugary drinks:** Water is the healthiest drink for your teeth and general wellness. If you do desire a sugary drink, consider a diet or sugar-free version.
- **Eat fruits and veggies instead of sugary snacks:** Fruits and vegetables are rich with vitamins, minerals, and antioxidants that are healthy for your teeth and general health.

- **Choose whole grains over processed grains:** Whole grains are a wonderful source of fibre, which may assist to clean teeth and gums.
- **Avoid sticky foods:** If you do consume sticky foods, be sure to clean your teeth promptly afterwards.
- **Eat hard foods with caution:** If you do consume hard items, be sure to bite them gently and avoid chewing on them with your front teeth.

By following these guidelines, you may minimise your consumption of foods that are unhealthy for your teeth and help to maintain your teeth healthy and strong for a lifetime.

Breakfast recipes

Here are some breakfast dishes for kids that are both tasty and beneficial for oral health:

Oatmeal with Berries and Nuts

Ingredients:

- 1/2 cup rolled oats

- 1 cup milk of choice

- 1/4 cup berries

- 1/4 cup nuts and seeds

Instructions:

Combine the oats and milk in a saucepan. Bring to a boil over medium heat. Reduce the heat to low and simmer for 5 minutes, or till the oats are cooked through. Stir in the berries, nuts, and seeds.

This oatmeal is a wonderful source of fibre, which may help clean teeth and gums. The berries and nuts also give crucial vitamins and minerals that are helpful for oral health.

Yogurt Parfait

Ingredients:

- 1 cup plain yoghourt

- 1/2 cup chopped fruit (such as berries, bananas, or apples)

- 1/4 cup granola

Instructions:

Layer the yoghurt, fruit, and granola in a jar or parfait glass.
Keep repeating the layers until the jar or glass is filled.

This parfait is a wonderful source of calcium, protein, and fibre. Calcium is vital for healthy teeth, protein helps to repair and rebuild gum tissue, and fibre helps to clean teeth and gums.

Smoothie

Ingredients:

- 1 cup milk of choice

- 1/2 cup fruit (such as berries, bananas, or yoghourt)

- 1 tablespoon honey or maple syrup (optional)

Instructions:

Mix all ingredients together in a blender and mix until smooth.
This smoothie is a wonderful source of calcium, protein, and vitamins. Calcium is

vital for healthy teeth, protein helps to repair and rebuild gum tissue, and vitamins are crucial for general health, including dental health.

Whole-wheat bread with avocado

Ingredients:

- 1 piece of whole wheat bread

- 1/4 avocado, mashed

- 1/4 teaspoon salt

- 1/4 teaspoon black pepper

Instructions:

Toast the bread.
Spread the mashed avocado on the bread.
Season with salt and pepper.
This toast is a fantastic source of fibre and healthy fats. Fibre helps to clean teeth and

gums, and healthy fats are crucial for general health, including dental health.

By following these recommendations, you may help your kid establish good eating habits that will last a lifetime.

Lunch recipes

Here are some lunch ideas for kids that are both tasty and beneficial for oral health:

Fruit and Yogurt Parfait

Ingredients:

- 1 cup plain yoghourt

- 1/2 cup chopped fruit (such as berries, bananas, or apples)

- 1/4 cup granola

Instructions:

Layer the yoghurt, fruit, and granola in a jar or parfait glass.
Repeat the layers till the jar or glass is filled.
This parfait is a wonderful source of calcium, protein, and fibre. Calcium is vital for healthy teeth, protein helps to repair and

rebuild gum tissue, and fibre helps to clean teeth and gums.

Veggie Quesadillas

Ingredients:

- 2 whole wheat tortillas

- 1/4 cup shredded cheese

- 1/4 cup chopped veggies (such as carrots, peppers, or onions)

Instructions:

Spread the cheese on one tortilla.
Top with the veggies.
Place the other tortilla on top.
Heat a lightly oiled skillet over average heat.
Place the quesadilla in the pan and cook for 1-2 minutes each side, or until the cheese is melted and the tortillas are golden brown.

These quesadillas are a wonderful source of fibre and vitamins. Fibre helps to clean teeth and gums, and vitamins are crucial for general health, including dental health.

Chicken Nuggets

Ingredients:

- 1 pound of ground chicken

- 1/2 cup bread crumbs

- 1/4 cup grated Parmesan cheese

- 1 egg, beaten

- 1/4 teaspoon salt

- 1/4 teaspoon black pepper

Instructions:

The oven should be Preheated to 400 degrees F (200 degrees C).
In a big bowl, add all the ingredients and stir thoroughly.
Shape the mixture into tiny nuggets.
Take the nugget and place it on a baking sheet lined with parchment paper.
Bake for 15-20 minutes, or till it is cooked through.
Serve with your favourite dipping sauce.

These chicken nuggets are a fantastic source of protein, which is vital for repairing and rebuilding gum tissue. They are also quite low in sugar, which is helpful for tooth health.

Smoothie

Ingredients:

- 1 cup milk of choice

- 1/2 cup fruit (such as berries, bananas, or yoghourt)

- 1 tablespoon honey or maple syrup (optional)

Instructions:

Mix all ingredients together in a blender and mix until smooth.
Serve and enjoy!

This smoothie is a wonderful source of calcium, protein, and vitamins. Calcium is vital for healthy teeth, protein helps to repair and rebuild gum tissue, and vitamins are crucial for general health, including dental health.

By making lunch entertaining and enticing, you may encourage your kids to consume nutritious dishes and snacks.

Dinner recipes

Dinner dishes for kids dental health:

Salmon with Roasted Vegetables

Salmon is an excellent source of omega-3 fatty acids, which are helpful for general health, including tooth health. Roasted veggies are a wonderful source of fibre and vitamins, which are also vital for tooth health.

Ingredients:

- 1 pound of salmon fillet

- 1 tablespoon olive oil

- 1/2 teaspoon salt

- 1/4 teaspoon black pepper

- 1 cup chopped veggies (such as carrots, broccoli, or zucchini)

Instructions:

The oven should be Preheated to 400 degrees F (200 degrees C).
Place the salmon fillet on a baking pan lined with parchment paper.
Drizzle olive oil, season with pepper and salt
Roast for 15-20 minutes, or till the fish is cooked through.
Serve with roasted veggies.

Chicken Stir-Fry

Chicken stir-fry is a fast and simple dish that is filled with nutrition. Chicken is a rich source of protein, which is vital for repairing and rebuilding gum tissue. Vegetables are a wonderful source of fibre and vitamins, which are also vital for oral health.

Ingredients:

- Cut 1 pound boneless skinless chicken breasts into strips

- 1 tablespoon vegetable oil

- 1 onion, chopped

- 1 green pepper, chopped

- 1 red pepper, chopped

- 1/4 cup soy sauce

- 1 tablespoon honey or maple syrup

- 1 tablespoon cornstarch

- 1/4 cup water

Instructions:

Heat the oil in a large skillet or wok over average heat.
Add the chicken and heat until browned on both sides.

Add the onion, peppers, soy sauce, honey, cornstarch, and water.

Bring to a boil, then reduce heat and simmer for 5 minutes, or till the sauce has thickened.

Serve over rice.

Lentil Soup

Lentil soup is a hearty and nutritious meal that is good for dental health. Lentils are a good source of fibre and protein, which are important for dental health. Vegetables are a wonderful source of fibre and vitamins, which are also vital for oral health.

Ingredients:

- 1 cup lentils

- 2 cups vegetable broth

- 1 onion, chopped

- 2 carrots, chopped

- 2 celery stalks, chopped

- 1 teaspoon garlic powder

- 1/2 teaspoon salt

- 1/4 teaspoon black pepper

Instructions:

Rinse the lentils in a sieve.
Combine the lentils, vegetable broth, onion, carrots, celery, garlic powder, salt, and pepper in a large saucepan.
Bring to a boil over medium heat.
Reduce the heat to low and simmer for 20–30 minutes, or until the lentils are cooked.
Serve and enjoy!

These are just a few examples of supper dishes that are healthy for kids' oral health. There are many more fantastic recipes accessible online and in cookbooks. When picking recipes, be careful to consider your child's nutritional requirements and preferences. You may also be creative and experiment with other tastes and ingredients.

By following these recommendations, you may help your kid establish good eating habits that will last a lifetime.

Snacks recipes

Snacks are a vital component of a child's diet, but they may also be a big source of sugar and bad fats. By selecting nutritious snacks, you may help your kid maintain excellent oral health and general wellness.

Here are some snack dishes that are both tasty and excellent for kids' oral health:

Fruit smoothie

Ingredients:

- 1 cup milk of choice

- 1 banana

- 1 cup berries

- 1 tablespoon honey or maple syrup (optional)

Instructions:

Combine all ingredients in a blender and mix till it is smooth.
Enjoy!

Fruit smoothies are a terrific method to urge youngsters to eat their fruits and veggies. They are also a wonderful source of calcium, protein, and vitamins, which are all vital for oral health.

Veggie quesadilla

Ingredients:

- 2 whole-wheat tortillas

- 1/4 cup shredded cheese

- 1/4 cup chopped veggies (such as carrots, bell peppers, or onions)

Instructions:

Spread the cheese on one tortilla.
Top with the veggies.
Place the other tortilla on top.
Heat a lightly oiled skillet over average heat.
Place the quesadilla in the pan and cook for
1-2 minutes each side, or until the cheese is
melted and the tortillas are golden brown.
Cut into quarters and enjoy!

Veggie quesadillas are a wonderful source of
fibre and vitamins, which are all vital for
tooth health. They are also a fun and quick
snack for youngsters to enjoy.

Trail mix

Ingredients:

- 1/2 cup of nuts (such as almonds,
  walnuts, or cashews)

- 1/2 cup seeds (such as pumpkin seeds, sunflower seeds, or chia seeds)

- 1/4 cup dried fruit (such as raisins, cranberries, or apricots)

Instructions:

Combine all ingredients in a bowl.
Enjoy!

Trail mix is a wonderful source of protein, fibre, and healthy fats, which are all necessary for oral health. It is also a handy snack that is convenient to carry on the run.

Yoghourt parfait

Ingredients:

- 1 cup plain yoghourt

- 1/2 cup chopped fruit (such as berries, bananas, or apples)

- 1/4 cup granola

Instructions:

Layer the yoghurt, fruit, and granola in a jar or parfait glass.
Repeat the layers till the jar or glass is filled.
Enjoy!

Yoghourt parfaits are a fantastic source of calcium, protein, and fibre, which are all vital for oral health. They are also a fun and simple snack for youngsters to create.

Hard-boiled eggs

Ingredients:

- 6 eggs

- 1/4 cup water

- 1/4 teaspoon salt

Instructions:

Put the egg into a single layer of saucepan
Add the water and salt.
Bring to a boil over high heat.
Cover and remove from heat.
Let it stand for 10 minutes.
Drain and run cold water over the eggs until
they are cool enough to handle.
Peel and enjoy!

Hard-boiled eggs are a fantastic source of protein, which is vital for repairing and rebuilding gum tissue. They are also a handy snack that is convenient to carry on the run.

These are just a few examples of snack dishes that are beneficial for kids' oral health. There are many more fantastic recipes accessible online and in cookbooks. When picking recipes, be careful to consider your child's nutritional requirements and preferences. You may also be creative and experiment with other tastes and ingredients.

By following these recommendations, you may help your kid establish good eating habits that will last a lifetime.

Chapter 3

Oral health care tips for kids

Oral health is vital for everyone, but it is particularly critical for youngsters. Their teeth and gums are still growing, and they are more prone to cavities and other dental disorders.

Here are some oral health care suggestions for kids:

- **Start cleaning their teeth early:** As soon as your child's first tooth comes in, start brushing it with a soft toothbrush and water. When your kid is two years old, you may start using a pea-sized quantity of fluoride toothpaste.
- **Brush their teeth twice a day for two minutes**: Make sure your youngster washes their teeth in the morning and before night. Help them

wash their teeth thoroughly, particularly the regions behind their teeth and around the gum line.

- **Floss their teeth once a day:** Flossing helps to eliminate plaque and food particles from between teeth, where a toothbrush cannot reach. Start flossing your child's teeth when they have two teeth that touch.
- **Take them to the dentist for regular checkups and cleanings:** It is crucial to take your kid to the dentist for frequent examinations and cleanings, even if they don't have any dental concerns. This will help prevent cavities and other dental issues from forming.

Here are some extra recommendations for helping your kid establish excellent dental health habits:

- **Make brushing and flossing entertaining:** Choose a fun toothbrush and toothpaste for your youngster. You may also sing songs or play games as they brush and floss.
- **Be a positive role model:** Brush and floss your teeth frequently in front of your youngster.
- **Limit sugary beverages and snacks:** Sugar is a primary food supply for bacteria in the mouth, which may contribute to cavities. Limit your child's consumption of sugary beverages and snacks, such as soda, juice, candy, and cookies.
- **Encourage them to drink lots of water:** Water helps to wipe away food particles and plaque from the teeth. Encourage your youngster to drink water throughout the day.

By following these guidelines, you may help your kid establish excellent dental health practices that will last a lifetime.ng their teeth early.

The important of regular dental check-ups

Regular dental check-ups are vital for everyone, but they are particularly critical for youngsters. Kids' teeth and gums are still growing, and they are more prone to cavities and other dental disorders.

Here are some of the reasons why frequent dental check-ups are vital for kids:

- **help discover and treat tooth issues early:** Early identification and treatment of oral disorders may help prevent more severe problems from occurring. For example, a tiny cavity may be simply filled, whereas a big cavity may need a more difficult operation, like a crown or root canal.
- **To monitor the growth of teeth and gums:** Dentists may examine to make sure that youngsters' teeth and gums are growing appropriately. They may also discover and address any

abnormalities early on, such as crooked teeth, overcrowding, or jaw difficulties.

- **To educate youngsters about proper dental hygiene routines:** Dentists can educate youngsters how to clean and floss their teeth correctly. They may also give recommendations on nutrition and lifestyle changes that can assist support excellent oral health.

Here are some of the advantages of frequent dental check-ups for kids:

- **Healthier teeth and gums:** Regular dental check-ups and cleanings may help maintain youngsters' teeth and gums healthy. This may help to avoid cavities, gum disease, and other oral issues.
- **Reduced pain and suffering:** Early identification and treatment of

dental disorders may assist to avoid pain and suffering. For example, a little hollow may be quickly filled without any discomfort, whereas a big cavity may need more difficult and unpleasant operations.

- **Decrease dental expenditures.** Early diagnosis and treatment of dental issues may help save money in the long term. For example, a tiny hollow may be quickly filled for a relatively modest cost, whereas a big cavity may need more sophisticated and costly operations.
- **More confidence:** A healthy grin may help youngsters feel more secure. Regular dental check-ups and cleanings may help youngsters attain and keep a healthy smile.

How frequently should kids go to the dentist?

The American Dental Association (ADA) advises that youngsters visit the dentist for a check-up and cleaning every six months. This is the greatest approach to ensure that their teeth and gums are healthy and that any dental issues are recognized and addressed early.

How to prepare your kid for a dental check-up

It is crucial to prepare your kid for their dental checkup. This will assist to lessen any anxiety they may have. Here are some tips:

- **Talk to your youngster about what to anticipate at the dentist's office:** Explain that the dentist will be looking at their teeth and gums and cleaning them.

- **Read books or watch videos on going to the dentist:** This might make your youngster feel more comfortable with the event.
- **Practice brushing and flossing your child's teeth together:** This will help them get acclimated to the sensation of having their teeth and gums cleaned.

Let your kid know that it is appropriate to ask questions and to let the dentist know if they are feeling uncomfortable.

By following these guidelines, you may help your kid have a great experience at the dentist's office. Regular dental check-ups are a crucial aspect of maintaining excellent oral health for youngsters.

Fun and educational activities for teaching oral care

Here are some entertaining and instructive exercises for teaching dental care to kids:

Make a tooth model.

This is a terrific method for youngsters to learn about the various components of a tooth and how to clean and floss correctly. You may use a number of materials to build a tooth model, such as clay, play dough, or even a hard-boiled egg.

Have a tooth-brushing party.

This is a fun and engaging approach to educate youngsters about the significance of cleaning their teeth. Gather up all of your child's favourite toothbrushes and toothpaste, then throw on some music. Then everyone may clean their teeth together. You may even create a game out of it and see who can wash their teeth the longest or the most completely.

Play brushing games.

There are many different brushing games that you may play with your youngster. For example, you may play a game where you see who can wash their teeth first, or you can play a game where you see who can clean their teeth without getting any toothpaste on their face.

Read literature on oral care.

There are many fantastic books available that educate youngsters about oral care. These books may be a fun and educational method to educate youngsters about the significance of cleaning and flossing their teeth.

Sing songs about oral care.

There are also numerous songs available that educate youngsters about dental care. These songs may be a fun and appealing method to educate youngsters about the significance of cleaning and flossing their teeth.

Visit the dentist.

Taking your kid to the dentist for regular examinations and cleanings is a terrific approach to educate them about the significance of dental care. The dentist may also address any questions that your kid may have regarding oral health.

Here are some extra ways for making dental care entertaining and instructive for kids:

- **Make it a routine:** Brush and floss your child's teeth with them every day. This will assist to build a schedule that they will be more likely to keep to when they become older.

- **Be positive:** Make oral care a pleasurable experience for your kid. Use engaging and entertaining words, and be sure you thank them for a good job.
- **Be creative:** There are many different methods to make dental care entertaining and informative for youngsters. Get imaginative and come up with fresh activities that your youngster will appreciate.

By following these guidelines, you may help your kid establish excellent dental health practices that will last a lifetime.

Conclusion

Conclusion of dental health cookbooks for kids

Dental health cookbooks for kids are a terrific method to educate children about the significance of eating healthy meals for their teeth and gums. They may also help make healthy eating entertaining and engaging for youngsters.

Here are some recommendations for utilising oral health recipes for kids:

- Choose cookbooks that are suitable for your child's age and interests.

- Involve your youngster in the cooking process. This will help kids learn about various cuisines and how to cook them.

- Make cooking entertaining for your youngster. Let them help you measure ingredients, mix batter, and decorate final meals.

- Serve the nutritious meals and snacks that you create together. This will let your toddler learn that nutritious meals can be delightful.

Dental·health cookbooks for kids may be a helpful tool for educating children about the significance of dental health. They may also help make healthy eating entertaining and engaging for youngsters. By following the guidelines above, you can utilise dental health cookbooks to help your kid build good eating habits that will last a lifetime.

In addition to the aforementioned, here are some more advice for parents:

- Make sure the recipes in the cookbook are fit for your child's dietary requirements and limitations.

- If your kid has any allergies or dietary sensitivities, be careful to alter the recipes appropriately.

- Be creative and experiment with various tastes and ingredients. This will assist to preserve your child's interest in healthy eating.

- Talk to your kid about the various foods they are consuming and why they are beneficial for their teeth and gums.

- Make sure your youngster is receiving adequate calcium and vitamin D in their diet. These nutrients are needed for good teeth and bones.

By following these recommendations, you can help your kid build a healthy connection with food and understand the significance of dental health.

www.ingramcontent.com/pod-product-compliance
Lightning Source LLC
Chambersburg PA
CBHW061007260726
48661CB00005B/2087

ISBN 9798864594780
90000
9 798864 594780

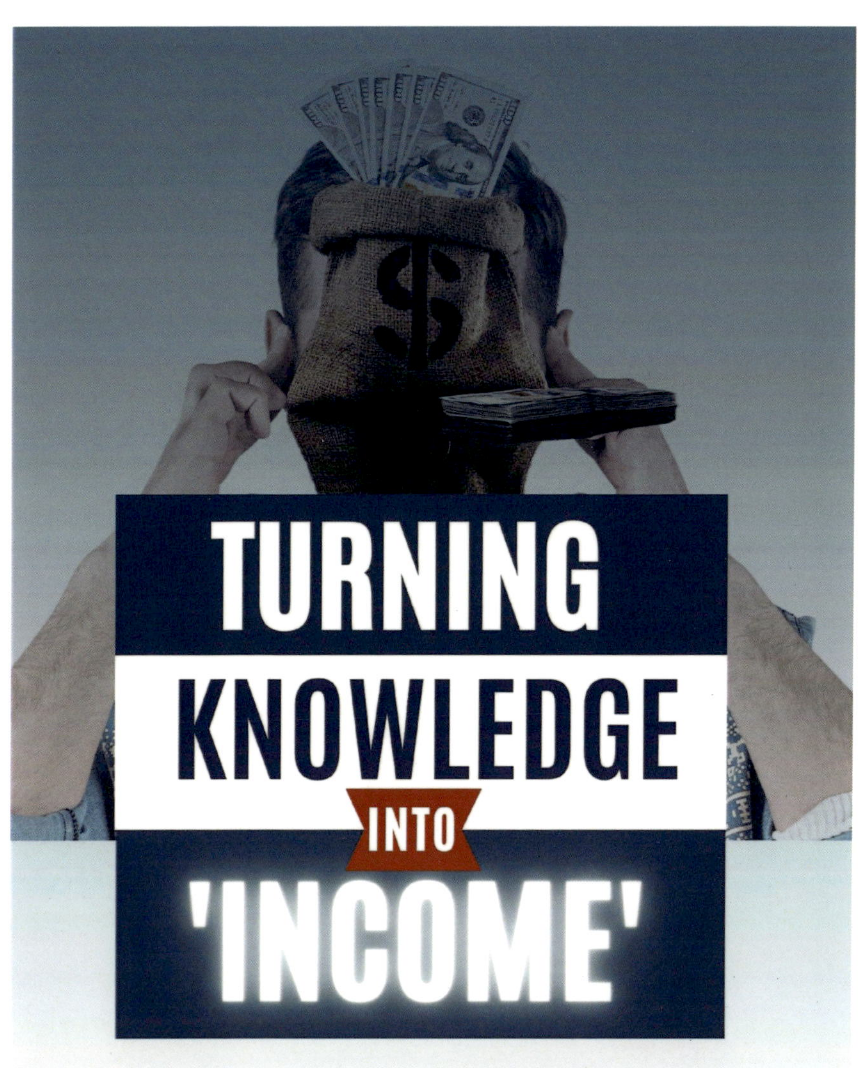

TURNING
KNOWLEDGE
INTO
'INCOME'
UNLOCKING EARNINGS FROM YOUR
INSIGHTS AND SKILLS
ROBERT J. WHITE